FOOD *AND* EXERCISE JOURNAL

WORK.
SWEAT.
REPEAT.

MY NAME

....

....

ISBN: 9781091960619

WEEK 1	1	2	3	4	5	6	7
WEEK 2	8	9	10	11	12	13	14
WEEK 3	15	16	17	18	19	20	21
WEEK 4	22	23	24	25	26	27	28
WEEK 5	29	30	31	32	33	34	35
WEEK 6	36	37	38	39	40	41	42
WEEK 7	43	44	45	46	47	48	49
WEEK 8	50	51	52	53	54	55	56
WEEK 9	57	58	59	60	61	62	63
WEEK 10	64	65	66	67	68	69	70
WEEK 11	71	72	73	74	75	76	77
WEEK 12	78	79	80	81	82	83	84
WEEK 13	85	86	87	88	89	90	

DAY 1

MY MEASUREMENTS

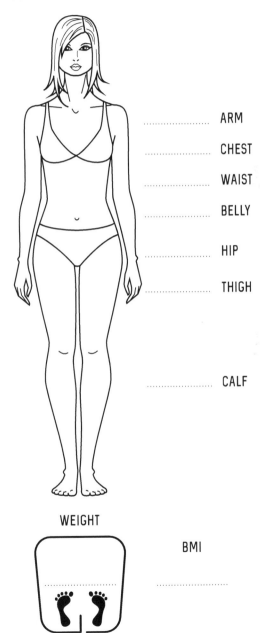

.... ARM

.... CHEST

.... WAIST

.... BELLY

.... HIP

.... THIGH

.... CALF

WEIGHT

BMI

....

DAY (1)

MO TU WE TH FR SA SU

DATE ....

HOW I FEEL

:D :) :| :(

BREAKFAST

....
....
....
....
....

SNACKS

....
....
....

TOTAL CALORIES

_____

PROTEIN CONTENT FIBER CONTENT

_____ _____

OTHER

....

LUNCH

....
....
....
....
....
....
....
....
....
....

DINNER

....
....
....
....
....
....
....
....
....
....

WEIGHT   SLEEP   WATER   PROTEIN

_____   _____

♥ EXERCISE / OTHER ACTIVITIES   SET / REPS / DISTANCE   TIME

....
....
....
....

NOTES

....
....

🕐 6A 7 8 9 10 11 12P 1 2 3 4 5 6 7 8 9 10+

B=BREAKFAST   L=LUNCH   D=DINNER   S=SNACKS   E=EXERCISE

HOW I FEEL

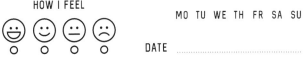

MO TU WE TH FR SA SU

DATE ....

DAY (2)

BREAKFAST

....
....
....
....
....
_____ __

SNACKS

....
....
....

TOTAL CALORIES

_____

PROTEIN CONTENT FIBER CONTENT

_____ _____

OTHER

....

LUNCH

....
....
....
....
....
....
....
....
....
....

DINNER

....
....
....
....
....
....
....
....
....
....

WEIGHT   SLEEP   WATER   PROTEIN

....

EXERCISE / OTHER ACTIVITIES | SET / REPS / DISTANCE | TIME

EXERCISE / OTHER ACTIVITIES	SET / REPS / DISTANCE	TIME
....	....	....
....	....	....
....	....	....
....	....	....
....	....	....

NOTES

....
....
....

6A 7 8 9 10 11 12P 1 2 3 4 5 6 7 8 9 10+

B=BREAKFAST   L=LUNCH   D=DINNER   S=SNACKS   E=EXERCISE

DAY (3)

MO TU WE TH FR SA SU

DATE ....

HOW I FEEL

BREAKFAST

LUNCH

DINNER

....
....
....
....
....

SNACKS

....
....
....

TOTAL CALORIES

PROTEIN CONTENT FIBER CONTENT

WEIGHT

SLEEP

WATER

PROTEIN

OTHER
....

♡ EXERCISE / OTHER ACTIVITIES

SET / REPS / DISTANCE

TIME

....
....
....
....

NOTES
....
....

6A 7 8 9 10 11 12P 1 2 3 4 5 6 7 8 9 10+

B=BREAKFAST   L=LUNCH   D=DINNER   S=SNACKS   E=EXERCISE

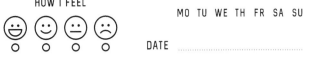

HOW I FEEL

MO TU WE TH FR SA SU

DATE ....

DAY ④

BREAKFAST

....
....
....
....
....
....

_____ ____

SNACKS

....
....
....

_____ ____

TOTAL CALORIES

_____

PROTEIN CONTENT   FIBER CONTENT

_____ _____

OTHER

....

LUNCH

....
....
....
....
....
....
....
....
....
....
....

DINNER

....
....
....
....
....
....

WEIGHT   **SLEEP**   **WATER**   **PROTEIN**

_____ _____ ....

EXERCISE / OTHER ACTIVITIES

SET / REPS / DISTANCE   TIME

....
....
....
....
....

NOTES

....
....

6A   7   8   9   10   11   12P   1   2   3   4   5   6   7   8   9   10+

B=BREAKFAST   L=LUNCH   D=DINNER   S=SNACKS   E=EXERCISE

DAY (5)

MO TU WE TH FR SA SU

DATE ....

BREAKFAST

....
....
....
....
....

_____ _____

SNACKS

....
....
....

_____ _____

LUNCH

....
....
....
....
....
....
....
....
....
....

DINNER

....
....
....
....
....
....
....
....
....

TOTAL CALORIES

_____

PROTEIN CONTENT   FIBER CONTENT

_____ _____

OTHER
....

WEIGHT   **SLEEP**   **WATER**   **PROTEIN**

============

♥ EXERCISE / OTHER ACTIVITIES

SET / REPS / DISTANCE   TIME

....
....
....
....
....

NOTES

....
....
....

🕐 6A 7 8 9 10 11 12P 1 2 3 4 5 6 7 8 9 10+

B=BREAKFAST   L=LUNCH   D=DINNER   S=SNACKS   E=EXERCISE

HOW I FEEL

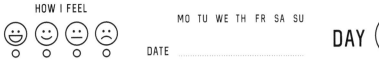

MO TU WE TH FR SA SU

DATE ....

DAY (6)

BREAKFAST
....
....
....
....
....
_____ _____

SNACKS
....
....
....

_____ _____

LUNCH
....
....
....
....
....
....
....
....
....

DINNER
....
....
....
....
....
....
....
....
....

TOTAL CALORIES
_____

PROTEIN CONTENT   FIBER CONTENT

_____ _____

OTHER
....

WEIGHT   **SLEEP**   **WATER**   **PROTEIN**

_____ _____   ....

♥ EXERCISE / OTHER ACTIVITIES

	SET / REPS / DISTANCE	TIME
....	....	....
....	....	....
....	....	....
....	....	....
....	....	....

NOTES
....
....

🕐 6A 7 8 9 10 11 12P 1 2 3 4 5 6 7 8 9 10+

B=BREAKFAST   L=LUNCH   D=DINNER   S=SNACKS   E=EXERCISE

DAY (7)

MO TU WE TH FR SA SU

DATE ....

HOW I FEEL

☺ ☺ ☺ ☹
○ ○ ○ ○

BREAKFAST
....
....
....
....
....
_____ ____

SNACKS
....
....
....

_____ ____

TOTAL CALORIES
_____

PROTEIN CONTENT FIBER CONTENT
_____ _____

OTHER
....

LUNCH
....
....
....
....
....
....
....
....
....
....

DINNER
....
....
....
....
....
....
....
....
....

WEIGHT SLEEP WATER PROTEIN
_____ ....

♥ EXERCISE / OTHER ACTIVITIES

SET / REPS / DISTANCE   TIME

....
....
....
....
....

NOTES
....
....

🕐 6A 7 8 9 10 11 12P 1 2 3 4 5 6 7 8 9 10+

B=BREAKFAST L=LUNCH D=DINNER S=SNACKS E=EXERCISE

HOW I FEEL

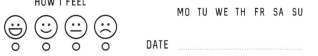

MO TU WE TH FR SA SU

DATE ....

DAY (8)

BREAKFAST
....
....
....
....
....
_____ _____

SNACKS
....
....
....
_____ _____

LUNCH
....
....
....
....
....
....
....
....
....
....
....
....

DINNER
....
....
....
....
....
....
....
....
....
....
....

TOTAL CALORIES
_____

PROTEIN CONTENT   FIBER CONTENT
_____ _____

OTHER
....

WEIGHT   SLEEP   WATER   PROTEIN

♥ EXERCISE / OTHER ACTIVITIES   SET / REPS / DISTANCE   TIME
....
....
....
....
....

NOTES
....
....

🕐 6A 7 8 9 10 11 12P 1 2 3 4 5 6 7 8 9 10+

B=BREAKFAST   L=LUNCH   D=DINNER   S=SNACKS   E=EXERCISE

DAY (9)

DATE ....

HOW I FEEL

😀 🙂 😐 🙁
○ ○ ○ ○

BREAKFAST

....
....
....
....
....

SNACKS

....
....
....

TOTAL CALORIES

_____

PROTEIN CONTENT   FIBER CONTENT

_____ _____

OTHER

....

LUNCH

....
....
....
....
....
....
....
....
....
....
....

DINNER

....
....
....
....
....
....
....
....
....

WEIGHT   **SLEEP**   **WATER**   **PROTEIN**

=====================   ....

❤ EXERCISE / OTHER ACTIVITIES

	SET / REPS / DISTANCE	TIME
....		....
....		....
....		....
....		....
....		....

NOTES

....
....

🕐 6A 7 8 9 10 11 12P 1 2 3 4 5 6 7 8 9 10+

B=BREAKFAST   L=LUNCH   D=DINNER   S=SNACKS   E=EXERCISE

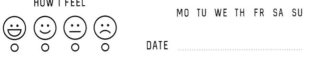

HOW I FEEL

MO TU WE TH FR SA SU

DATE ....

DAY (10)

BREAKFAST

....
....
....
....
....
_____ ____

SNACKS

....
....
....
_____ ____

TOTAL CALORIES

_____

PROTEIN CONTENT   FIBER CONTENT

_____ _____

OTHER

....

LUNCH

....
....
....
....
....
....
....
....
....
....
....
....

DINNER

....
....
....
....
....
....
....
....
....
....
....

WEIGHT   **SLEEP**   **WATER**   **PROTEIN**

_____   _____   ....

EXERCISE / OTHER ACTIVITIES	SET / REPS / DISTANCE	TIME
....	....	....
....	....	....
....	....	....
....	....	....
....	....	....

NOTES

....
....

6A 7 8 9 10 11 12P 1 2 3 4 5 6 7 8 9 10+

B=BREAKFAST   L=LUNCH   D=DINNER   S=SNACKS   E=EXERCISE

DAY (11)

DATE ....

HOW I FEEL

BREAKFAST

LUNCH

DINNER

....

....

....

....

....

_____ _____

SNACKS

....

....

....

TOTAL CALORIES

_____

PROTEIN CONTENT   FIBER CONTENT

WEIGHT   SLEEP   WATER   PROTEIN

_____ _____

OTHER

....

♥ EXERCISE / OTHER ACTIVITIES   SET / REPS / DISTANCE   TIME

....

....

....

....

....

NOTES

....

....

6A 7 8 9 10 11 12P 1 2 3 4 5 6 7 8 9 10+

B=BREAKFAST   L=LUNCH   D=DINNER   S=SNACKS   E=EXERCISE

HOW I FEEL

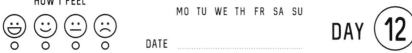

MO TU WE TH FR SA SU

DATE ....

DAY (12)

BREAKFAST

....
....
....
....
....

SNACKS

....
....
....

TOTAL CALORIES

PROTEIN CONTENT FIBER CONTENT

OTHER
....

LUNCH

....
....
....
....
....
....
....
....
....
....
....

WEIGHT   SLEEP   WATER   PROTEIN

DINNER

....
....
....
....
....
....
....
....
....
....
....

EXERCISE / OTHER ACTIVITIES   SET / REPS / DISTANCE   TIME

....
....
....
....
....

NOTES

....
....
....

6A 7 8 9 10 11 12P 1 2 3 4 5 6 7 8 9 10+

B=BREAKFAST   L=LUNCH   D=DINNER   S=SNACKS   E=EXERCISE

DAY (13)

DATE ....

HOW I FEEL

BREAKFAST   LUNCH   DINNER

SNACKS

TOTAL CALORIES

WEIGHT   SLEEP   WATER   PROTEIN

PROTEIN CONTENT   FIBER CONTENT

OTHER

EXERCISE / OTHER ACTIVITIES   SET / REPS / DISTANCE   TIME

NOTES

6A 7 8 9 10 11 12P 1 2 3 4 5 6 7 8 9 10+

B=BREAKFAST   L=LUNCH   D=DINNER   S=SNACKS   E=EXERCISE

HOW I FEEL

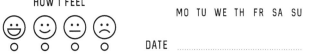

MO TU WE TH FR SA SU

DATE ....

DAY (14)

BREAKFAST	LUNCH	DINNER
....	....	....
....	....	....
....	....	....
....	....	....
....	....	....

SNACKS
....
....
....
....

TOTAL CALORIES
_____

PROTEIN CONTENT   FIBER CONTENT

WEIGHT   SLEEP   WATER   PROTEIN

OTHER
....

♡ EXERCISE / OTHER ACTIVITIES   SET / REPS / DISTANCE   TIME

....
....
....
....
....

NOTES
....
....

🕐 6A 7 8 9 10 11 12P 1 2 3 4 5 6 7 8 9 10+

B=BREAKFAST   L=LUNCH   D=DINNER   S=SNACKS   E=EXERCISE

DAY (15)

DATE ....

HOW I FEEL

BREAKFAST   LUNCH   DINNER

....
....
....
....
....
_____ ___   ....

SNACKS   ....
....
....
....
_____ ___   ....

TOTAL CALORIES

WEIGHT   SLEEP   WATER   PROTEIN

_____

PROTEIN CONTENT FIBER CONTENT

_____ ___   _____ ....

OTHER
....

♥ EXERCISE / OTHER ACTIVITIES   SET / REPS / DISTANCE   TIME

....
....
....
....
_____   _____ _____

NOTES
....
....

🕐 6A 7 8 9 10 11 12P 1 2 3 4 5 6 7 8 9 10+

B=BREAKFAST L=LUNCH D=DINNER S=SNACKS E=EXERCISE

HOW I FEEL

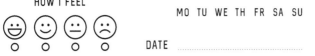

MO TU WE TH FR SA SU

DATE ....

DAY (16)

BREAKFAST

LUNCH

DINNER

....

....

....

....

....

SNACKS

....

....

....

TOTAL CALORIES

_____

WEIGHT   SLEEP   WATER   PROTEIN

PROTEIN CONTENT   FIBER CONTENT

OTHER

....

♡ EXERCISE / OTHER ACTIVITIES   SET / REPS / DISTANCE   TIME

....

....

....

....

....

NOTES

....

....

🕐 6A 7 8 9 10 11 12P 1 2 3 4 5 6 7 8 9 10+

B=BREAKFAST   L=LUNCH   D=DINNER   S=SNACKS   E=EXERCISE

DAY (17)

DATE ....

HOW I FEEL

☺ ☺ ☺ ☹
○ ○ ○ ○

BREAKFAST
....
....
....
....
....

SNACKS
....
....
....

TOTAL CALORIES
_____

PROTEIN CONTENT   FIBER CONTENT
_____ _____

LUNCH
....
....
....
....
....
....
....
....

DINNER
....
....
....
....
....
....
....
....

WEIGHT   SLEEP   WATER   PROTEIN

OTHER
....
....

❤ EXERCISE / OTHER ACTIVITIES   SET / REPS / DISTANCE   TIME
....
....
....
....
....

NOTES
....
....
....

| 6A | 7 | 8 | 9 | 10 | 11 | 12P | 1 | 2 | 3 | 4 | 5 | 6 | 7 | 8 | 9 | 10+ |

B=BREAKFAST   L=LUNCH   D=DINNER   S=SNACKS   E=EXERCISE

HOW I FEEL

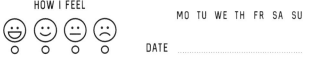

MO TU WE TH FR SA SU

DATE ....

DAY (18)

BREAKFAST

....
....
....
....
....

_____ ____

SNACKS

....
....
....

TOTAL CALORIES

_____ ____

PROTEIN CONTENT   FIBER CONTENT

_____ ____

OTHER

....

LUNCH

....
....
....
....
....
....
....
....
....
....
....

WEIGHT   SLEEP   WATER   PROTEIN

DINNER

....
....
....
....
....
....
....
....
....
....
....

❤ EXERCISE / OTHER ACTIVITIES   SET / REPS / DISTANCE   TIME

....
....
....
....
....
                                          _____ _____

NOTES

....
....
....

🕐 6A 7 8 9 10 11 12P 1 2 3 4 5 6 7 8 9 10+

B=BREAKFAST   L=LUNCH   D=DINNER   S=SNACKS   E=EXERCISE

DAY (19)

DATE ....

HOW I FEEL

😃 ○ 🙂 ○ 😐 ○ 🙁 ○

BREAKFAST
....
....
....
....
....
_____ ___

LUNCH
....
....
....
....
....
....

DINNER
....
....
....
....
....
....

SNACKS
....
....
....
....
_____ ___

TOTAL CALORIES
_____

PROTEIN CONTENT   FIBER CONTENT
_____ _____

WEIGHT   SLEEP   WATER   PROTEIN

OTHER
....
....

❤ EXERCISE / OTHER ACTIVITIES

SET / REPS / DISTANCE   TIME

....
....
....
....
....

NOTES
....
....
....

🕐 6A 7 8 9 10 11 12P 1 2 3 4 5 6 7 8 9 10+

B=BREAKFAST   L=LUNCH   D=DINNER   S=SNACKS   E=EXERCISE

HOW I FEEL

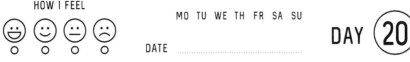

MO TU WE TH FR SA SU

DATE ....

DAY 20

BREAKFAST

....
....
....
....
....

SNACKS

....
....
....

TOTAL CALORIES

_____

PROTEIN CONTENT FIBER CONTENT

_____   _____

OTHER

....

LUNCH

....
....
....
....
....
....
....
....
....
....

DINNER

....
....
....
....
....
....
....
....
....

WEIGHT   **SLEEP**   **WATER**   **PROTEIN**

♥ EXERCISE / OTHER ACTIVITIES

	SET / REPS / DISTANCE	TIME
....	....	....
....	....	....
....	....	....
....	....	....
....	....	....

NOTES

....
....

6A 7 8 9 10 11 12P 1 2 3 4 5 6 7 8 9 10+

B=BREAKFAST L=LUNCH D=DINNER S=SNACKS E=EXERCISE

DAY (21)

HOW I FEEL

BREAKFAST

....
....
....
....
....
....

_____ _____

SNACKS

....
....
....

TOTAL CALORIES

_____ _____

PROTEIN CONTENT FIBER CONTENT

_____ _____

OTHER
....

LUNCH

....
....
....
....
....
....
....
....
....
....

DINNER

....
....
....
....
....
....
....
....
....
....

WEIGHT   SLEEP   WATER   PROTEIN

♥ EXERCISE / OTHER ACTIVITIES

EXERCISE / OTHER ACTIVITIES	SET / REPS / DISTANCE	TIME
....		....
....		....
....		....
....		....
....		....

NOTES

....
....

6A 7 8 9 10 11 12P 1 2 3 4 5 6 7 8 9 10+

B=BREAKFAST   L=LUNCH   D=DINNER   S=SNACKS   E=EXERCISE

HOW I FEEL

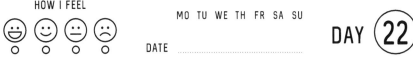

MO TU WE TH FR SA SU

DATE ....

DAY (22)

BREAKFAST

....
....
....
....
....

_____ __

SNACKS

....
....
....

_____ ___

LUNCH

....
....
....
....
....
....
....
....
....
....

DINNER

....
....
....
....
....

TOTAL CALORIES

_____

PROTEIN CONTENT FIBER CONTENT

_____ _____

OTHER

....

WEIGHT   SLEEP   WATER   PROTEIN

EXERCISE / OTHER ACTIVITIES

SET / REPS / DISTANCE   TIME

....
....
....
....
....
....

NOTES

....
....
....

6A 7 8 9 10 11 12P 1 2 3 4 5 6 7 8 9 10+

B=BREAKFAST   L=LUNCH   D=DINNER   S=SNACKS   E=EXERCISE

DAY (23)

MO TU WE TH FR SA SU

DATE ....

HOW I FEEL

☺ ☺ ☺ ☹
○   ○   ○   ○

BREAKFAST

....
....
....
....
....
_____ ____

SNACKS

....
....
....
....
_____ ____

TOTAL CALORIES

_____ ____

PROTEIN CONTENT FIBER CONTENT

_____ ____

OTHER

....

LUNCH

....
....
....
....
....
....
....
....
....
....

DINNER

....
....
....
....
....
....
....
....
....

WEIGHT   SLEEP   WATER   PROTEIN

_____ _____ ....

♥ EXERCISE / OTHER ACTIVITIES   SET / REPS / DISTANCE   TIME

.... | .... | ....
.... | .... | ....
.... | .... | ....
.... | .... | ....
_____ | _____ | _____

NOTES

....
....
....

🕐 6A 7 8 9 10 11 12P 1 2 3 4 5 6 7 8 9 10+

B=BREAKFAST L=LUNCH D=DINNER S=SNACKS E=EXERCISE

HOW I FEEL

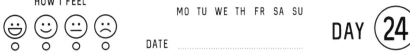

MO TU WE TH FR SA SU

DATE ....

DAY ㉔

BREAKFAST

....
....
....
....
....
_____   _____

SNACKS

....
....
....

TOTAL CALORIES

_____

PROTEIN CONTENT FIBER CONTENT

_____   _____   _____

OTHER

....

LUNCH

....
....
....
....
....
....
....
....
....
....
....

DINNER

....
....
....
....
....
....
....
....
....
....

WEIGHT	SLEEP	WATER	PROTEIN

EXERCISE / OTHER ACTIVITIES

EXERCISE / OTHER ACTIVITIES	SET / REPS / DISTANCE	TIME
....	....	....
....	....	....
....	....	....
....	....	....
....	....	....

NOTES

....
....
....

6A	7	8	9	10	11	12P	1	2	3	4	5	6	7	8	9	10+

B=BREAKFAST   L=LUNCH   D=DINNER   S=SNACKS   E=EXERCISE

DAY (25)

DATE ....

HOW I FEEL

😃 🙂 😐 ☹
○ ○ ○ ○

BREAKFAST

....
....
....
....
....
_____ ____

SNACKS

....
....
....
_____ ____

LUNCH

....
....
....
....
....
....
....

DINNER

....
....
....
....
....
....
....

TOTAL CALORIES

_____

PROTEIN CONTENT FIBER CONTENT

_____ ____

WEIGHT   SLEEP   WATER   PROTEIN

OTHER
....

❤ EXERCISE / OTHER ACTIVITIES

	SET / REPS / DISTANCE	TIME
....		....
....		....
....		....
....		....
....		....

NOTES

....
....

🕐 6A 7 8 9 10 11 12P 1 2 3 4 5 6 7 8 9 10+

B=BREAKFAST L=LUNCH D=DINNER S=SNACKS E=EXERCISE

HOW I FEEL

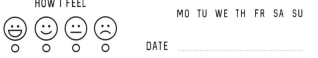

MO TU WE TH FR SA SU

DATE ....

DAY (26)

BREAKFAST

....
....
....
....
....

SNACKS

....
....
....
....

LUNCH

....
....
....
....
....
....
....
....
....
....
....
....

DINNER

....
....
....
....
....
....
....
....
....
....
....
....

TOTAL CALORIES

_____

PROTEIN CONTENT   FIBER CONTENT

_____   _____

OTHER

....

WEIGHT   **SLEEP**   **WATER**   **PROTEIN**

♥ EXERCISE / OTHER ACTIVITIES

SET / REPS / DISTANCE   TIME

.... | .... | ....
.... | .... | ....
.... | .... | ....
.... | .... | ....
.... | .... | ....

NOTES

....
....
....

🕐 6A 7 8 9 10 11 12P 1 2 3 4 5 6 7 8 9 10+

B=BREAKFAST   L=LUNCH   D=DINNER   S=SNACKS   E=EXERCISE

DAY (27)

DATE ....

HOW I FEEL

BREAKFAST

LUNCH

DINNER

SNACKS

TOTAL CALORIES

WEIGHT

SLEEP

WATER

PROTEIN

PROTEIN CONTENT   FIBER CONTENT

OTHER

EXERCISE / OTHER ACTIVITIES

SET / REPS / DISTANCE

TIME

NOTES

6A 7 8 9 10 11 12P 1 2 3 4 5 6 7 8 9 10+

B=BREAKFAST   L=LUNCH   D=DINNER   S=SNACKS   E=EXERCISE

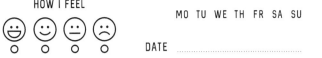

HOW I FEEL

MO TU WE TH FR SA SU

DATE ....

DAY (28)

BREAKFAST
....
....
....
....
....
_____ _____

SNACKS
....
....
....

TOTAL CALORIES
_____

PROTEIN CONTENT FIBER CONTENT
_____ _____

OTHER
....

LUNCH
....
....
....
....
....
....
....
....
....
....
....
....

DINNER
....
....
....
....
....
....
....
....

WEIGHT   SLEEP   WATER   PROTEIN
_____ _____ ....

EXERCISE / OTHER ACTIVITIES   SET / REPS / DISTANCE   TIME
....
....
....
....
....
_____   _____   _____

NOTES
....
....
....

6A 7 8 9 10 11 12P 1 2 3 4 5 6 7 8 9 10+

B=BREAKFAST   L=LUNCH   D=DINNER   S=SNACKS   E=EXERCISE

DAY (29)

MO TU WE TH FR SA SU

DATE ....

HOW I FEEL

BREAKFAST

....
....
....
....
....
_____ ___

SNACKS

....
....
....
_____ ___

TOTAL CALORIES
_____

PROTEIN CONTENT FIBER CONTENT
_____ _____

OTHER
....

LUNCH

....
....
....
....
....
....
....
....
....
_____ ___

WEIGHT

_____

DINNER

....
....
....
....
....
....
....
....
....
_____ ___

SLEEP   WATER   PROTEIN
....

EXERCISE / OTHER ACTIVITIES   SET / REPS / DISTANCE   TIME

....
....
....
....
....
_____   _____   _____

NOTES
....
....
....

6A 7 8 9 10 11 12P 1 2 3 4 5 6 7 8 9 10+
B=BREAKFAST   L=LUNCH   D=DINNER   S=SNACKS   E=EXERCISE

DAY 30

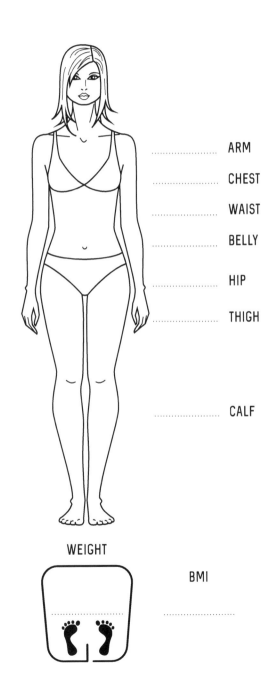

ARM ....

CHEST ....

WAIST ....

BELLY ....

HIP ....

THIGH ....

CALF ....

WEIGHT

BMI

DAY (30)

MO TU WE TH FR SA SU

DATE ....

HOW I FEEL

BREAKFAST   LUNCH   DINNER

....
....
....
....
....
_____ ___   ....

SNACKS   ....
....
....
....
_____ ___   ....

TOTAL CALORIES

_____   WEIGHT   SLEEP   WATER   PROTEIN

PROTEIN CONTENT FIBER CONTENT

_____ _____   ========

OTHER
....

♡ EXERCISE / OTHER ACTIVITIES   SET / REPS / DISTANCE   TIME

....
....
....
....
....

NOTES
....
....

🕐 6A 7 8 9 10 11 12P 1 2 3 4 5 6 7 8 9 10+
B=BREAKFAST   L=LUNCH   D=DINNER   S=SNACKS   E=EXERCISE

HOW I FEEL

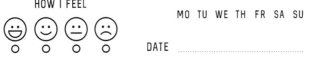

MO TU WE TH FR SA SU

DATE ....

DAY (31)

BREAKFAST

....
....
....
....
....
_____ ____

SNACKS

....
....
....

TOTAL CALORIES

_____

PROTEIN CONTENT FIBER CONTENT

_____ _____

OTHER

....

LUNCH

....
....
....
....
....
....
....
....
....
....
....

DINNER

....
....
....
....
....
....
....
....
....
....

WEIGHT   SLEEP   WATER   PROTEIN

EXERCISE / OTHER ACTIVITIES

	SET / REPS / DISTANCE	TIME
....	....	....
....	....	....
....	....	....
....	....	....
....	....	....

NOTES

....
....

6A 7   8   9   10 11 12P 1   2   3   4   5   6   7   8   9   10+

B=BREAKFAST   L=LUNCH   D=DINNER   S=SNACKS   E=EXERCISE

DAY (32)

DATE ....

HOW I FEEL

:D :) :| :(
O   O   O   O

BREAKFAST

....
....
....
....
....
_____ ____

SNACKS

....
....
....
_____ ____

TOTAL CALORIES
_____

PROTEIN CONTENT FIBER CONTENT
_____ _____

OTHER
....

LUNCH

....
....
....
....
....

....
....
....

DINNER

....
....
....
....
....

....
....
....

WEIGHT **SLEEP** **WATER** **PROTEIN**

....

EXERCISE / OTHER ACTIVITIES	SET / REPS / DISTANCE	TIME
....	....	....
....	....	....
....	....	....
....	....	....
....	....	....

NOTES

....
....

6A 7 8 9 10 11 12P 1 2 3 4 5 6 7 8 9 10+

B=BREAKFAST L=LUNCH D=DINNER S=SNACKS E=EXERCISE

HOW I FEEL

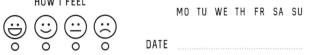

MO TU WE TH FR SA SU

DATE ....

DAY (33)

BREAKFAST

....
....
....
....
....

_____ _____

SNACKS

....
....
....
....

LUNCH

....
....
....
....
....
....
....
....
....
....

DINNER

....
....
....
....
....
....
....
....
....
....

TOTAL CALORIES

_____

PROTEIN CONTENT FIBER CONTENT

_____ _____

OTHER

....

WEIGHT	SLEEP	WATER	PROTEIN

EXERCISE / OTHER ACTIVITIES   SET / REPS / DISTANCE   TIME

....
....
....
....
....
....

NOTES

....
....
....

6A 7 8 9 10 11 12P 1 2 3 4 5 6 7 8 9 10+

B=BREAKFAST   L=LUNCH   D=DINNER   S=SNACKS   E=EXERCISE

DAY (34)

MO TU WE TH FR SA SU

DATE ....

HOW I FEEL

:D :) :| :(
O   O   O   O

BREAKFAST

....
....
....
....
....
_____ ____

SNACKS

....
....
....
_____ ____

TOTAL CALORIES

_____

PROTEIN CONTENT FIBER CONTENT

_____ _____

OTHER

....

LUNCH

....
....
....
....
....
....
....
....
....
....
_____ ____

DINNER

....
....
....
....
....
....
....
....
....
....
_____ ____

WEIGHT   SLEEP   WATER   PROTEIN

_____ _____ ....

EXERCISE / OTHER ACTIVITIES

	SET / REPS / DISTANCE	TIME
....	....	....
....	....	....
....	....	....
....	....	....
....	....	....

NOTES

....
....

6A 7 8 9 10 11 12P 1 2 3 4 5 6 7 8 9 10+

B=BREAKFAST   L=LUNCH   D=DINNER   S=SNACKS   E=EXERCISE

HOW I FEEL

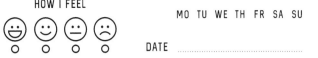

MO TU WE TH FR SA SU

DATE ....

DAY (35)

BREAKFAST

....
....
....
....
....

SNACKS

....
....
....

TOTAL CALORIES

_____

PROTEIN CONTENT   FIBER CONTENT

_____   _____

OTHER
....

LUNCH

....
....
....
....
....
....
....
....
....
....

DINNER

....
....
....
....
....
....
....
....

WEIGHT   SLEEP   WATER   PROTEIN

_____ _____ ....

♡ EXERCISE / OTHER ACTIVITIES

SET / REPS / DISTANCE   TIME

....
....
....
....
....

NOTES

....
....

| 6A | 7 | 8 | 9 | 10 | 11 | 12P | 1 | 2 | 3 | 4 | 5 | 6 | 7 | 8 | 9 | 10+ |

B=BREAKFAST   L=LUNCH   D=DINNER   S=SNACKS   E=EXERCISE

DAY (36)

MO TU WE TH FR SA SU

DATE ....

HOW I FEEL

:D :) :| :(

BREAKFAST

....
....
....
....
....
_____ ___

SNACKS

....
....
....
....
_____ ___

TOTAL CALORIES

_____ ___

PROTEIN CONTENT   FIBER CONTENT

_____ ___

OTHER

....

LUNCH

....
....
....
....
....
....
....
....
....
....

DINNER

....
....
....
....
....
....
....
....
....
....

WEIGHT   **SLEEP**   **WATER**   **PROTEIN**

EXERCISE / OTHER ACTIVITIES

	SET / REPS / DISTANCE	TIME
....	....	....
....	....	....
....	....	....
....	....	....
....	....	....

NOTES

....
....
....

6A 7 8 9 10 11 12P 1 2 3 4 5 6 7 8 9 10+

B=BREAKFAST   L=LUNCH   D=DINNER   S=SNACKS   E=EXERCISE

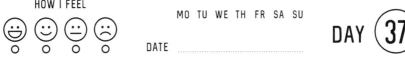

HOW I FEEL

MO TU WE TH FR SA SU

DATE ....

DAY (37)

BREAKFAST

....
....
....
....
....

LUNCH

DINNER

SNACKS

....
....
....

TOTAL CALORIES

_____

PROTEIN CONTENT FIBER CONTENT

_____ _____

WEIGHT

SLEEP

WATER

PROTEIN

OTHER

....

♡ **EXERCISE / OTHER ACTIVITIES**   SET / REPS / DISTANCE   TIME

....
....
....
....
....

NOTES

....
....
....

🕐 6A 7 8 9 10 11 12P 1 2 3 4 5 6 7 8 9 10+

B=BREAKFAST   L=LUNCH   D=DINNER   S=SNACKS   E=EXERCISE

DAY (38)

DATE ....

HOW I FEEL

😄 ○ 🙂 ○ 😐 ○ ☹️ ○

BREAKFAST

....
....
....
....
....
_____ _____

SNACKS

....
....
....
_____ _____

TOTAL CALORIES

_____

PROTEIN CONTENT   FIBER CONTENT
_____ _____

OTHER

....

LUNCH

....
....
....
....
....
....
....
....
....
....

DINNER

....
....
....
....
....
....
....
....
....

WEIGHT   SLEEP   WATER   PROTEIN

....

❤️ EXERCISE / OTHER ACTIVITIES

	SET / REPS / DISTANCE	TIME
....		
....		
....		
....		
....		

NOTES

....
....

  6A 7 8 9 10 11 12P 1 2 3 4 5 6 7 8 9 10+

B=BREAKFAST   L=LUNCH   D=DINNER   S=SNACKS   E=EXERCISE

HOW I FEEL

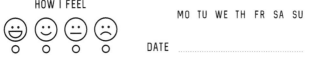

MO TU WE TH FR SA SU

DATE ....

DAY (39)

BREAKFAST

....
....
....
....
....
_____ _____

SNACKS

....
....
....

LUNCH

....
....
....
....
....
....
....
....
....
....

DINNER

....
....
....
....
....
....
....
....
....
....

TOTAL CALORIES
_____

PROTEIN CONTENT FIBER CONTENT
_____ _____

WEIGHT

SLEEP

WATER

PROTEIN

OTHER
....

EXERCISE / OTHER ACTIVITIES   SET / REPS / DISTANCE   TIME

....
....
....
....
....

NOTES

....
....

6A 7 8 9 10 11 12P 1 2 3 4 5 6 7 8 9 10+

B=BREAKFAST L=LUNCH D=DINNER S=SNACKS E=EXERCISE

DAY (40)

DATE ....

HOW I FEEL

BREAKFAST

....
....
....
....
....
_____ ___

SNACKS

....
....
....
_____ ___

TOTAL CALORIES
_____

PROTEIN CONTENT FIBER CONTENT
_____ ___

OTHER
....

LUNCH

....
....
....
....
....
....
....
....
....
....

DINNER

....
....
....
....
....
....
....
....
....

WEIGHT   SLEEP   WATER   PROTEIN

❤ EXERCISE / OTHER ACTIVITIES   SET / REPS / DISTANCE   TIME

....
....
....
....
....

NOTES

....
....

6A 7 8 9 10 11 12P 1 2 3 4 5 6 7 8 9 10+

B=BREAKFAST   L=LUNCH   D=DINNER   S=SNACKS   E=EXERCISE

HOW I FEEL

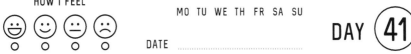

MO TU WE TH FR SA SU

DATE ....

DAY (41)

BREAKFAST

....
....
....
....
....

_____ _____

SNACKS

....
....
....
....

_____ _____

LUNCH

....
....
....
....
....
....
....
....
....
....
....
....

DINNER

....
....
....
....
....
....
....
....
....
....
....
....

TOTAL CALORIES

_____

PROTEIN CONTENT FIBER CONTENT

_____ _____

WEIGHT **SLEEP** **WATER** **PROTEIN**

=====

OTHER

....

EXERCISE / OTHER ACTIVITIES   SET / REPS / DISTANCE   TIME

....
....
....
....
....
....

_____ _____ _____

NOTES

....
....
....

6A 7 8 9 10 11 12P 1 2 3 4 5 6 7 8 9 10+

B=BREAKFAST L=LUNCH D=DINNER S=SNACKS E=EXERCISE

DAY (42)

MO TU WE TH FR SA SU

DATE ....

HOW I FEEL

😄 ○ 🙂 ○ 😐 ○ 🙁 ○

BREAKFAST

....
....
....
....
....

SNACKS

....
....
....

TOTAL CALORIES

PROTEIN CONTENT   FIBER CONTENT

OTHER

....

LUNCH

....
....
....
....
....
....
....
....
....
....

DINNER

....
....
....
....
....
....
....
....
....
....

WEIGHT   SLEEP   WATER   PROTEIN

♡ EXERCISE / OTHER ACTIVITIES   SET / REPS / DISTANCE   TIME

....
....
....
....
....

NOTES

....
....

6A 7 8 9 10 11 12P 1 2 3 4 5 6 7 8 9 10+

B=BREAKFAST   L=LUNCH   D=DINNER   S=SNACKS   E=EXERCISE

HOW I FEEL

MO TU WE TH FR SA SU

DATE ....

DAY 43

BREAKFAST	LUNCH	DINNER
....	....	....
....	....	....
....	....	....
....	....	....
....	....	....

SNACKS

....

....

....

TOTAL CALORIES

_____

PROTEIN CONTENT   FIBER CONTENT

_____   _____

WEIGHT   SLEEP   WATER   PROTEIN

OTHER

....

EXERCISE / OTHER ACTIVITIES   SET / REPS / DISTANCE   TIME

....

....

....

....

NOTES

....

....

6A 7 8 9 10 11 12P 1 2 3 4 5 6 7 8 9 10+

B=BREAKFAST   L=LUNCH   D=DINNER   S=SNACKS   E=EXERCISE

DAY (44)

MO TU WE TH FR SA SU

DATE ....

HOW I FEEL

BREAKFAST
....
....
....
....
....
_____ _____

SNACKS
....
....
....
_____ _____

TOTAL CALORIES
_____

PROTEIN CONTENT   FIBER CONTENT
_____ _____

OTHER
....

LUNCH
....
....
....
....
....
....
....
....
....

DINNER
....
....
....
....
....
....
....
....
....

WEIGHT   SLEEP   WATER   PROTEIN
_____

♡ EXERCISE / OTHER ACTIVITIES   SET / REPS / DISTANCE   TIME
....
....
....
....
....
_____   _____   _____

NOTES
....
....
....

6A 7 8 9 10 11 12P 1 2 3 4 5 6 7 8 9 10+

B=BREAKFAST   L=LUNCH   D=DINNER   S=SNACKS   E=EXERCISE

HOW I FEEL

☺ ☺ ☺ ☹
○ ○ ○ ○

MO TU WE TH FR SA SU

DATE ....

DAY (45)

BREAKFAST   LUNCH   DINNER

....

....

....

....

....

_____   ___

SNACKS   ....

....

....

....

TOTAL CALORIES   WEIGHT   SLEEP   WATER   PROTEIN
_____

PROTEIN CONTENT FIBER CONTENT

_____ ___   _____   ....

OTHER

....

♡ EXERCISE / OTHER ACTIVITIES   SET / REPS / DISTANCE   TIME

....

....

....

....

....

NOTES

....

....

🕐 6A 7 8 9 10 11 12P 1 2 3 4 5 6 7 8 9 10+

B=BREAKFAST   L=LUNCH   D=DINNER   S=SNACKS   E=EXERCISE

DAY (46)

MO TU WE TH FR SA SU

DATE ....

HOW I FEEL

BREAKFAST

LUNCH

DINNER

SNACKS

TOTAL CALORIES

WEIGHT   SLEEP   WATER   PROTEIN

PROTEIN CONTENT   FIBER CONTENT

OTHER

♥ EXERCISE / OTHER ACTIVITIES   SET / REPS / DISTANCE   TIME

NOTES

🕐   6A   7   8   9   10   11   12P   1   2   3   4   5   6   7   8   9   10+

B=BREAKFAST   L=LUNCH   D=DINNER   S=SNACKS   E=EXERCISE

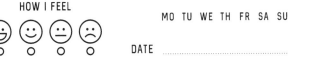

HOW I FEEL

MO TU WE TH FR SA SU

DATE ....

DAY (47)

BREAKFAST
....
....
....
....
....
_____ _____

SNACKS
....
....
....
_____ _____

LUNCH
....
....
....
....
....
....
....
....
....
....

DINNER
....
....
....
....
....

TOTAL CALORIES
_____

PROTEIN CONTENT FIBER CONTENT
_____ _____

WEIGHT   SLEEP   WATER   PROTEIN
_____ _____ ....

OTHER
....

♥ EXERCISE / OTHER ACTIVITIES

SET / REPS / DISTANCE   TIME

....
....
....
....
_____ _____ _____

NOTES
....
....

6A 7 8 9 10 11 12P 1 2 3 4 5 6 7 8 9 10+

B=BREAKFAST   L=LUNCH   D=DINNER   S=SNACKS   E=EXERCISE

DAY (48)

DATE ....

HOW I FEEL

:D :) :| :(
O   O   O   O

BREAKFAST	LUNCH	DINNER
....	....	....
....	....	....
....	....	....
....	....	....
....	....	....

SNACKS

....
....
....

TOTAL CALORIES

_____

PROTEIN CONTENT   FIBER CONTENT

_____   _____

WEIGHT   SLEEP   WATER   PROTEIN

OTHER

....

♥ EXERCISE / OTHER ACTIVITIES   SET / REPS / DISTANCE   TIME

.... | .... | ....
.... | .... | ....
.... | .... | ....
.... | .... | ....

NOTES

....
....

🕐 6A 7 8 9 10 11 12P 1 2 3 4 5 6 7 8 9 10+

B=BREAKFAST   L=LUNCH   D=DINNER   S=SNACKS   E=EXERCISE

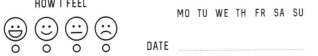

HOW I FEEL

MO TU WE TH FR SA SU

DATE ....

DAY 49

BREAKFAST

....
....
....
....
....
_____ _____

SNACKS

....
....
....

LUNCH

DINNER

TOTAL CALORIES

_____

PROTEIN CONTENT FIBER CONTENT

_____ _____ _____

WEIGHT   SLEEP   WATER   PROTEIN

OTHER

....

❤ EXERCISE / OTHER ACTIVITIES

SET / REPS / DISTANCE   TIME

....
....
....
....
....

NOTES

....
....

6A   7   8   9   10   11   12P   1   2   3   4   5   6   7   8   9   10+

B=BREAKFAST   L=LUNCH   D=DINNER   S=SNACKS   E=EXERCISE

DAY (50)

DATE ....

HOW I FEEL

😄   🙂   😐   🙁
○   ○   ○   ○

BREAKFAST

....
....
....
....
....

SNACKS

....
....
....

TOTAL CALORIES

_____

PROTEIN CONTENT   FIBER CONTENT

_____   _____

OTHER

....

LUNCH

....
....
....
....
....
....
....
....
....

DINNER

....
....
....
....
....
....
....
....

WEIGHT   SLEEP   WATER   PROTEIN
_____   _____   ....

♥ EXERCISE / OTHER ACTIVITIES

	SET / REPS / DISTANCE	TIME
....	....	....
....	....	....
....	....	....
....	....	....
....	....	....

NOTES

....
....

🕐 6A 7 8 9 10 11 12P 1 2 3 4 5 6 7 8 9 10+

B=BREAKFAST   L=LUNCH   D=DINNER   S=SNACKS   E=EXERCISE

HOW I FEEL

MO TU WE TH FR SA SU

DATE ....

DAY (51)

BREAKFAST

....
....
....
....
....
_____   _____

SNACKS

....
....
....

LUNCH

....
....
....
....
....
....
....
....
....

DINNER

....
....
....
....
....
....
....
....
....

TOTAL CALORIES

_____

PROTEIN CONTENT FIBER CONTENT

_____ _____

WEIGHT	SLEEP	WATER	PROTEIN

_____ ....

OTHER

....

❤ EXERCISE / OTHER ACTIVITIES

	SET / REPS / DISTANCE	TIME
....	....	....
....	....	....
....	....	....
....	....	....
....	....	....

NOTES

....
....
....

6A 7 8 9 10 11 12P 1 2 3 4 5 6 7 8 9 10+

B=BREAKFAST   L=LUNCH   D=DINNER   S=SNACKS   E=EXERCISE

DAY (52)

MO TU WE TH FR SA SU

DATE ....

HOW I FEEL

:D :) :| :(

BREAKFAST

....
....
....
....
....
_____

SNACKS

....
....
....

TOTAL CALORIES

_____

PROTEIN CONTENT **FIBER CONTENT**

_____ _____

LUNCH

....
....
....
....
....
....
....
....
....
....

DINNER

....
....
....
....
....
....
....
....
....
....

WEIGHT **SLEEP** **WATER** **PROTEIN**

_____ _____ ....

OTHER

....

♥ **EXERCISE / OTHER ACTIVITIES**   **SET / REPS / DISTANCE**   **TIME**

....
....
....
....
....

NOTES

....
....

6A 7 8 9 10 11 12P 1 2 3 4 5 6 7 8 9 10+

B=BREAKFAST L=LUNCH D=DINNER S=SNACKS E=EXERCISE

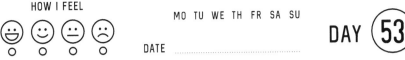

HOW I FEEL

MO TU WE TH FR SA SU

DATE ....

DAY (53)

BREAKFAST

....
....
....
....
....

LUNCH

....
....
....
....
....
....

DINNER

....
....
....
....
....

SNACKS

....
....
....

TOTAL CALORIES

_____

PROTEIN CONTENT   FIBER CONTENT

_____   _____

OTHER

....

WEIGHT   SLEEP   WATER   PROTEIN

....

EXERCISE / OTHER ACTIVITIES

SET / REPS / DISTANCE   TIME

....
....
....
....
....

NOTES

....
....

6A 7 8 9 10 11 12P 1 2 3 4 5 6 7 8 9 10+

B=BREAKFAST   L=LUNCH   D=DINNER   S=SNACKS   E=EXERCISE

DAY (54)

MO TU WE TH FR SA SU

DATE ....

HOW I FEEL

☺ ☺ ☺ ☹
○ ○ ○ ○

BREAKFAST

....
....
....
....
....

SNACKS

....
....
....

TOTAL CALORIES

_____

PROTEIN CONTENT   FIBER CONTENT

_____   _____

OTHER

....

LUNCH

....
....
....
....
....
....
....
....
....
....

DINNER

....
....
....
....
....
....
....
....
....

WEIGHT   **SLEEP**   **WATER**   **PROTEIN**

♡ **EXERCISE / OTHER ACTIVITIES**   SET / REPS / DISTANCE   TIME

....
....
....
....
....

NOTES

....
....

🕐 6A   7   8   9   10   11   12P   1   2   3   4   5   6   7   8   9   10+

B=BREAKFAST   L=LUNCH   D=DINNER   S=SNACKS   E=EXERCISE

HOW I FEEL

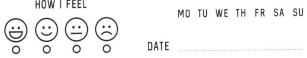

MO TU WE TH FR SA SU

DATE ....

DAY (55)

BREAKFAST

....
....
....
....
....

SNACKS

....
....
....

TOTAL CALORIES

_____

PROTEIN CONTENT FIBER CONTENT

_____ _____

OTHER

....

LUNCH

....
....
....
....
....
....
....
....
....
....
....
....

DINNER

....
....
....
....
....
....
....

WEIGHT **SLEEP** **WATER** **PROTEIN**

♥ EXERCISE / OTHER ACTIVITIES

SET / REPS / DISTANCE   TIME

....
....
....
....

NOTES

....
....

🕐 6A 7 8 9 10 11 12P 1 2 3 4 5 6 7 8 9 10+

B=BREAKFAST L=LUNCH D=DINNER S=SNACKS E=EXERCISE

DAY (56)

DATE ....

HOW I FEEL

😃 ☺️ 😐 ☹️
○   ○   ○   ○

BREAKFAST

LUNCH

DINNER

....
....
....
....
....

‾‾‾‾‾‾‾‾   ‾‾‾‾

SNACKS

....
....
....

TOTAL CALORIES

‾‾‾‾‾‾‾‾‾‾‾‾‾‾‾

PROTEIN CONTENT   FIBER CONTENT

‾‾‾‾‾‾‾   ‾‾‾‾‾

WEIGHT   SLEEP   WATER   PROTEIN

OTHER

‾‾‾‾‾‾‾‾‾   ....

....

❤ EXERCISE / OTHER ACTIVITIES

SET / REPS / DISTANCE   TIME

....
....
....
....
....

NOTES

....
....

🕐 6A 7 8 9 10 11 12P 1 2 3 4 5 6 7 8 9 10+

B=BREAKFAST   L=LUNCH   D=DINNER   S=SNACKS   E=EXERCISE

HOW I FEEL

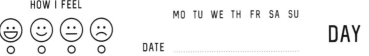

MO TU WE TH FR SA SU

DATE ....

DAY (57)

BREAKFAST

....
....
....
....
....
_____ ___

SNACKS

....
....
....
_____ ___

LUNCH

....
....
....
....
....
....
....
....
....
....
....
....

DINNER

....
....
....
....
....
....
....
....
....
....
....

TOTAL CALORIES

_____

PROTEIN CONTENT   FIBER CONTENT

_____   _____

OTHER

....

WEIGHT **SLEEP** **WATER** **PROTEIN**

_____ _____ ....

♡ EXERCISE / OTHER ACTIVITIES

	SET / REPS / DISTANCE	TIME
....	....	....
....	....	....
....	....	....
....	....	....
....	....	....

NOTES

....
....

 6A 7 8 9 10 11 12P 1 2 3 4 5 6 7 8 9 10+

B=BREAKFAST   L=LUNCH   D=DINNER   S=SNACKS   E=EXERCISE

DAY (58)

MO TU WE TH FR SA SU

DATE ....

HOW I FEEL

☺ ☺ ☺ ☹
○ ○ ○ ○

BREAKFAST

....
....
....
....
....
_____ _____

SNACKS

....
....
....

TOTAL CALORIES
_____

PROTEIN CONTENT   FIBER CONTENT
_____ _____

OTHER
....

LUNCH

....
....
....
....
....
....
....
....
....

DINNER

....
....
....
....
....
....
....
....

WEIGHT   **SLEEP**   **WATER**   **PROTEIN**
_____ ....

♡ **EXERCISE / OTHER ACTIVITIES**   SET / REPS / DISTANCE   TIME

....
....
....
....
....

NOTES

....
....

🕐 6A 7 8 9 10 11 12P 1 2 3 4 5 6 7 8 9 10+

B=BREAKFAST   L=LUNCH   D=DINNER   S=SNACKS   E=EXERCISE

HOW I FEEL

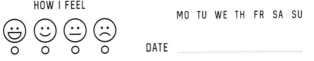

MO TU WE TH FR SA SU

DATE ....

DAY (59)

BREAKFAST

LUNCH

DINNER

SNACKS

TOTAL CALORIES

WEIGHT

SLEEP

WATER

PROTEIN

PROTEIN CONTENT FIBER CONTENT

OTHER

EXERCISE / OTHER ACTIVITIES

SET / REPS / DISTANCE

TIME

NOTES

6A 7 8 9 10 11 12P 1 2 3 4 5 6 7 8 9 10+

B=BREAKFAST   L=LUNCH   D=DINNER   S=SNACKS   E=EXERCISE

DAY 60

ARM ....

CHEST ....

WAIST ....

BELLY ....

HIP ....

THIGH ....

CALF ....

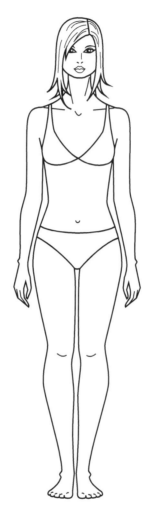

WEIGHT

BMI

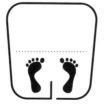

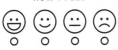

HOW I FEEL

MO TU WE TH FR SA SU

DATE ....

DAY 60

BREAKFAST

LUNCH

DINNER

SNACKS

TOTAL CALORIES

WEIGHT   SLEEP   WATER   PROTEIN

PROTEIN CONTENT FIBER CONTENT

OTHER

EXERCISE / OTHER ACTIVITIES   SET / REPS / DISTANCE   TIME

NOTES

6A 7 8 9 10 11 12P 1 2 3 4 5 6 7 8 9 10+

B=BREAKFAST   L=LUNCH   D=DINNER   S=SNACKS   E=EXERCISE

DAY (61)

MO TU WE TH FR SA SU

DATE ....

HOW I FEEL

☺ ☺ ☺ ☹
○ ○ ○ ○

BREAKFAST

....
....
....
....
....
....

_____ _____

SNACKS

....
....
....
....

TOTAL CALORIES

_____

PROTEIN CONTENT FIBER CONTENT

_____ _____

OTHER
....

LUNCH

....
....
....
....
....
....
....
....
....
....

DINNER

....
....
....
....
....
....
....
....
....

WEIGHT   SLEEP   WATER   PROTEIN

....

♥ EXERCISE / OTHER ACTIVITIES

	SET / REPS / DISTANCE	TIME
....	....	....
....	....	....
....	....	....
....	....	....
....	....	....

NOTES

....
....
....

🕐 6A 7 8 9 10 11 12P 1 2 3 4 5 6 7 8 9 10+

B=BREAKFAST L=LUNCH D=DINNER S=SNACKS E=EXERCISE

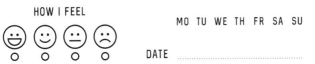

HOW I FEEL

MO TU WE TH FR SA SU

DATE ....

DAY 62

BREAKFAST

....
....
....
....
....

SNACKS

....
....
....

LUNCH

....
....
....
....
....
....
....
....
....
....
....

DINNER

....
....
....
....
....
....
....
....
....

TOTAL CALORIES

PROTEIN CONTENT   FIBER CONTENT

WEIGHT   SLEEP   WATER   PROTEIN

OTHER
....

EXERCISE / OTHER ACTIVITIES

SET / REPS / DISTANCE   TIME

NOTES

....
....

6A   7   8   9   10   11   12P   1   2   3   4   5   6   7   8   9   10+

B=BREAKFAST   L=LUNCH   D=DINNER   S=SNACKS   E=EXERCISE

DAY (63)

MO TU WE TH FR SA SU

DATE ....

HOW I FEEL

:D :) :| :(
O   O   O   O

BREAKFAST

....
....
....
....
....
_____

SNACKS

....
....
....
_____

TOTAL CALORIES
_____

PROTEIN CONTENT FIBER CONTENT
_____ _____

OTHER
....

LUNCH

....
....
....
....
....
....
....

DINNER

....
....
....
....

WEIGHT SLEEP WATER PROTEIN

♥ EXERCISE / OTHER ACTIVITIES

	SET / REPS / DISTANCE	TIME
....	....	....
....	....	....
....	....	....
....	....	....

NOTES

....
....

 6A 7 8 9 10 11 12P 1 2 3 4 5 6 7 8 9 10+

B=BREAKFAST L=LUNCH D=DINNER S=SNACKS E=EXERCISE

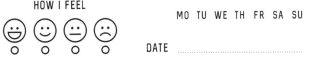

HOW I FEEL

MO TU WE TH FR SA SU

DATE ....

DAY 64

BREAKFAST
....
....
....
....
....
_____ __

SNACKS
....
....
....

LUNCH
....
....
....
....
....
....
....
....
....
....

DINNER
....
....
....
....
....
....
....
....
....
....

TOTAL CALORIES
_____

PROTEIN CONTENT FIBER CONTENT
_____ _____

WEIGHT   **SLEEP**   **WATER**   **PROTEIN**

OTHER
....

EXERCISE / OTHER ACTIVITIES

SET / REPS / DISTANCE   TIME

....
....
....
....
....

NOTES
....
....

6A 7 8 9 10 11 12P 1 2 3 4 5 6 7 8 9 10+

B=BREAKFAST L=LUNCH D=DINNER S=SNACKS E=EXERCISE

DAY (65)

DATE ....

HOW I FEEL

☺ ☺ ☺ ☹
○ ○ ○ ○

BREAKFAST

....
....
....
....
....
—————————— ——

SNACKS

....
....
....
—————————— ——

LUNCH

....
....
....
....
....
....
....
....

DINNER

....
....
....
....
....
....
....

TOTAL CALORIES

——————————————

PROTEIN CONTENT FIBER CONTENT
———————— ————————

WEIGHT   **SLEEP**   **WATER**   **PROTEIN**

OTHER

....
....

♥ EXERCISE / OTHER ACTIVITIES

	SET / REPS / DISTANCE	TIME
....	....	....
....	....	....
....	....	....
....	....	....

NOTES

....
....

🕐 6A 7 8 9 10 11 12P 1 2 3 4 5 6 7 8 9 10+

B=BREAKFAST L=LUNCH D=DINNER S=SNACKS E=EXERCISE

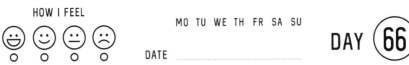

HOW I FEEL

MO TU WE TH FR SA SU

DATE ....

DAY 66

BREAKFAST

....
....
....
....
....

SNACKS

....
....
....

TOTAL CALORIES

_____

PROTEIN CONTENT FIBER CONTENT

_____ _____

OTHER

....

LUNCH

....
....
....
....
....
....
....
....
....
....
....

DINNER

....
....
....
....
....
....
....
....
....
....
....

WEIGHT   SLEEP   WATER   PROTEIN

♥ EXERCISE / OTHER ACTIVITIES   SET / REPS / DISTANCE   TIME

....
....
....
....
....

NOTES

....
....

6A   7   8   9   10   11   12P   1   2   3   4   5   6   7   8   9   10+

B=BREAKFAST   L=LUNCH   D=DINNER   S=SNACKS   E=EXERCISE

DAY (67)

MO TU WE TH FR SA SU

DATE ....

HOW I FEEL

BREAKFAST

....
....
....
....
....

_____   ____

SNACKS

....
....
....

TOTAL CALORIES

_____

PROTEIN CONTENT   FIBER CONTENT

_____   _____

OTHER

....

LUNCH

....
....
....
....
....
....
....
....
....

_____   ____

DINNER

....
....
....
....
....
....
....
....

_____

WEIGHT   SLEEP   WATER   PROTEIN

♥ EXERCISE / OTHER ACTIVITIES   SET / REPS / DISTANCE   TIME

....
....
....
....
....

NOTES

....
....

🕐 6A 7 8 9 10 11 12P 1 2 3 4 5 6 7 8 9 10+

B=BREAKFAST   L=LUNCH   D=DINNER   S=SNACKS   E=EXERCISE

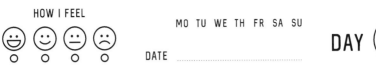

HOW I FEEL

MO TU WE TH FR SA SU

DATE ....

DAY 68

BREAKFAST

LUNCH

DINNER

SNACKS

TOTAL CALORIES

WEIGHT   SLEEP   WATER   PROTEIN

PROTEIN CONTENT FIBER CONTENT

OTHER

EXERCISE / OTHER ACTIVITIES   SET / REPS / DISTANCE   TIME

NOTES

6A 7 8 9 10 11 12P 1 2 3 4 5 6 7 8 9 10+

B=BREAKFAST   L=LUNCH   D=DINNER   S=SNACKS   E=EXERCISE

DAY (69)

HOW I FEEL

BREAKFAST

....
....
....
....
....
....
——————————   ———

SNACKS

....
....
....
——————————   ———

TOTAL CALORIES

——————————————

PROTEIN CONTENT FIBER CONTENT
———————— ————

OTHER
....

LUNCH

....
....
....
....
....

DINNER

....
....
....
....
....

WEIGHT   SLEEP   WATER   PROTEIN

❤ EXERCISE / OTHER ACTIVITIES   SET / REPS / DISTANCE   TIME

....
....
....
....
....

NOTES

....
....

6A 7 8 9 10 11 12P 1 2 3 4 5 6 7 8 9 10+

B=BREAKFAST   L=LUNCH   D=DINNER   S=SNACKS   E=EXERCISE

HOW I FEEL

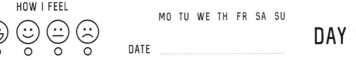

MO TU WE TH FR SA SU

DATE ....

DAY (70)

BREAKFAST
....
....
....
....
....
....

SNACKS
....
....
....

TOTAL CALORIES
_____

PROTEIN CONTENT   FIBER CONTENT
_____   _____

LUNCH
....
....
....
....
....
....
....
....
....
....

DINNER
....
....
....
....
....
....
....
....
....

WEIGHT   **SLEEP**   **WATER**   **PROTEIN**

_____ ....

OTHER
....

♥ EXERCISE / OTHER ACTIVITIES

	SET / REPS / DISTANCE	TIME
....	....	....
....	....	....
....	....	....
....	....	....
....	....	....

NOTES
....
....

🕐 6A 7 8 9 10 11 12P 1 2 3 4 5 6 7 8 9 10+

B=BREAKFAST   L=LUNCH   D=DINNER   S=SNACKS   E=EXERCISE

DAY (71)

MO TU WE TH FR SA SU

DATE ....

HOW I FEEL

☺ ☺ ☺ ☹
○ ○ ○ ○

BREAKFAST

....
....
....
....
....
_____ ___

SNACKS

....
....
....
_____ ___

LUNCH

....
....
....
....
....
....
....
....
....
....

DINNER

....
....
....
....
....
....
....
....
....
....

TOTAL CALORIES
_____

PROTEIN CONTENT   FIBER CONTENT
_____ ___

WEIGHT

SLEEP

WATER

PROTEIN

OTHER
....

♥ EXERCISE / OTHER ACTIVITIES

	SET / REPS / DISTANCE	TIME
....	....	....
....	....	....
....	....	....
....	....	....
....	....	....

NOTES

....
....

🕐 6A 7 8 9 10 11 12P 1 2 3 4 5 6 7 8 9 10+

B=BREAKFAST   L=LUNCH   D=DINNER   S=SNACKS   E=EXERCISE

HOW I FEEL

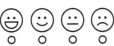

MO TU WE TH FR SA SU

DATE ....

DAY (72)

BREAKFAST

....
....
....
....
....

SNACKS

....
....
....

TOTAL CALORIES

_____

PROTEIN CONTENT   FIBER CONTENT

_____ _____

OTHER

....

LUNCH

....
....
....
....
....
....
....
....
....
....

DINNER

....
....
....
....
....
....

WEIGHT   SLEEP   WATER   PROTEIN

❤ **EXERCISE / OTHER ACTIVITIES**   SET / REPS / DISTANCE   TIME

....
....
....
....

NOTES

....
....

 6A 7 8 9 10 11 12P 1 2 3 4 5 6 7 8 9 10+

B=BREAKFAST   L=LUNCH   D=DINNER   S=SNACKS   E=EXERCISE

DAY (73)

MO TU WE TH FR SA SU

DATE ....

HOW I FEEL

:D   :)   :| :(
O   O   O   O

BREAKFAST

....
....
....
....
....

SNACKS

....
....
....

TOTAL CALORIES

_____

PROTEIN CONTENT   FIBER CONTENT

_____   _____

OTHER

....

LUNCH

....
....
....
....
....
....
....
....
....
....

WEIGHT   **SLEEP**   **WATER**   **PROTEIN**

....

DINNER

....
....
....
....
....
....
....
....
....

♥ EXERCISE / OTHER ACTIVITIES

SET / REPS / DISTANCE   TIME

....
....
....
....
....

NOTES

....
....

🕐 6A 7 8 9 10 11 12P 1 2 3 4 5 6 7 8 9 10+

B=BREAKFAST   L=LUNCH   D=DINNER   S=SNACKS   E=EXERCISE

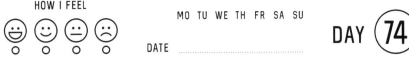

HOW I FEEL

MO TU WE TH FR SA SU

DATE ....

DAY (74)

BREAKFAST

....
....
....
....
....
_____ _____

SNACKS

....
....
....
....

LUNCH

DINNER

TOTAL CALORIES

_____

PROTEIN CONTENT FIBER CONTENT

_____ _____

OTHER

....

WEIGHT

SLEEP

WATER

PROTEIN

♥ EXERCISE / OTHER ACTIVITIES

SET / REPS / DISTANCE

TIME

NOTES

....
....

6A 7 8 9 10 11 12P 1 2 3 4 5 6 7 8 9 10+

B=BREAKFAST   L=LUNCH   D=DINNER   S=SNACKS   E=EXERCISE

DAY (75)

MO TU WE TH FR SA SU

DATE ....

HOW I FEEL

☺ 🙂 😐 ☹
○   ○   ○   ○

BREAKFAST

....
....
....
....
....
_____ ___

SNACKS

....
....
....
_____ ___

LUNCH

....
....
....
....
....
....
....
....
....
....

DINNER

....
....
....
....
....
....
....
....

TOTAL CALORIES
_____

PROTEIN CONTENT FIBER CONTENT
_____ _____

OTHER
....
....

WEIGHT **SLEEP** **WATER** **PROTEIN**

♥ EXERCISE / OTHER ACTIVITIES

	SET / REPS / DISTANCE	TIME
....	....	....
....	....	....
....	....	....
....	....	....
....	....	....

NOTES
....
....
....

🕐 6A 7 8 9 10 11 12P 1 2 3 4 5 6 7 8 9 10+

B=BREAKFAST L=LUNCH D=DINNER S=SNACKS E=EXERCISE

HOW I FEEL

MO TU WE TH FR SA SU

DATE ....

DAY (76)

BREAKFAST	LUNCH	DINNER
....	....	....
....	....	....
....	....	....
....	....	....
....	....	....
_____ __	....	....

SNACKS
.... | | .... | .... |

....

....

....

_____ __

TOTAL CALORIES

_____

PROTEIN CONTENT FIBER CONTENT

_____ _____

OTHER

....

....

WEIGHT   SLEEP   WATER   PROTEIN

♡ EXERCISE / OTHER ACTIVITIES

	SET / REPS / DISTANCE	TIME
....	....	....
....	....	....
....	....	....
....	....	....
....	....	....

NOTES

....

....

6A 7 8 9 10 11 12P 1 2 3 4 5 6 7 8 9 10+

B=BREAKFAST L=LUNCH D=DINNER S=SNACKS E=EXERCISE

DAY (77)

HOW I FEEL

😃 ◯ 🙂 ◯ 😐 ◯ 🙁 ◯

BREAKFAST

....
....
....
....
....
_____

SNACKS

....
....
....
_____

TOTAL CALORIES

_____

PROTEIN CONTENT   FIBER CONTENT

_____   _____

OTHER
....

LUNCH

....
....
....
....
....
....
....
....
....
....

DINNER

....
....
....
....
....
....
....
....
....

WEIGHT   SLEEP   WATER   PROTEIN

_____   _____   ....

❤ EXERCISE / OTHER ACTIVITIES   SET / REPS / DISTANCE   TIME

....
....
....
....
....

NOTES

....
....

🕐 | 6A | 7 | 8 | 9 | 10 | 11 | 12P | 1 | 2 | 3 | 4 | 5 | 6 | 7 | 8 | 9 | 10+

B=BREAKFAST   L=LUNCH   D=DINNER   S=SNACKS   E=EXERCISE

HOW I FEEL

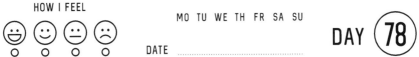

MO TU WE TH FR SA SU

DATE ....

DAY (78)

BREAKFAST
....
....
....
....
....
_____ ____

SNACKS
....
....
....

TOTAL CALORIES
_____

PROTEIN CONTENT FIBER CONTENT
_____ ____

OTHER
....

LUNCH
....
....
....
....
....
....
....
....
....
....
....
_____

DINNER
....
....
....
....
....
....
....
....

WEIGHT

SLEEP

WATER

PROTEIN

_____

❤ EXERCISE / OTHER ACTIVITIES

SET / REPS / DISTANCE

TIME

....
....
....
....
....

NOTES
....
....

🕐 6A 7 8 9 10 11 12P 1 2 3 4 5 6 7 8 9 10+

B=BREAKFAST L=LUNCH D=DINNER S=SNACKS E=EXERCISE

DAY (79)

MO TU WE TH FR SA SU

DATE ....

HOW I FEEL

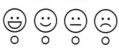

BREAKFAST

....
....
....
....
....

———————— ———

SNACKS

....
....
....

———————— ———

TOTAL CALORIES

————————————

PROTEIN CONTENT FIBER CONTENT

———————— ———

LUNCH

....
....
....
....
....
....
....
....
....

DINNER

....
....
....
....
....

WEIGHT   SLEEP   WATER   PROTEIN

————————————

OTHER

....

EXERCISE / OTHER ACTIVITIES   SET / REPS / DISTANCE   TIME

....
....
....
....
....

NOTES

....
....
....

6A 7 8 9 10 11 12P 1 2 3 4 5 6 7 8 9 10+

B=BREAKFAST L=LUNCH D=DINNER S=SNACKS E=EXERCISE

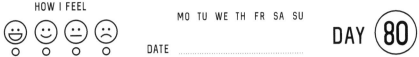

HOW I FEEL

MO TU WE TH FR SA SU

DATE ....

DAY (80)

BREAKFAST
....
....
....
....
....
_____ ____

SNACKS
....
....
....

TOTAL CALORIES
_____

PROTEIN CONTENT FIBER CONTENT
_____ ____ ____

OTHER
....

LUNCH
....
....
....
....
....
....
....
....
....
....
....

DINNER
....
....
....
....
....
....
....
....
....
....

WEIGHT   SLEEP   WATER   PROTEIN

♥ EXERCISE / OTHER ACTIVITIES

	SET / REPS / DISTANCE	TIME

NOTES
....
....

6A 7 8 9 10 11 12P 1 2 3 4 5 6 7 8 9 10+

B=BREAKFAST L=LUNCH D=DINNER S=SNACKS E=EXERCISE

DAY (81)

DATE ....

HOW I FEEL

😄 🙂 😐 🙁
○ ○ ○ ○

BREAKFAST
....
....
....
....
....
_____ ____

SNACKS
....
....
....
_____ ____

TOTAL CALORIES
_____

PROTEIN CONTENT FIBER CONTENT
_____ ____

OTHER
....

LUNCH
....
....
....
....
....
....
....
....
....

DINNER
....
....
....
....
....
....
....
....

WEIGHT   SLEEP   WATER   PROTEIN
_____ _____ ....

♥ EXERCISE / OTHER ACTIVITIES

	SET / REPS / DISTANCE	TIME
....		
....		
....		
....		
....		

NOTES
....
....

🕐 6A 7 8 9 10 11 12P 1 2 3 4 5 6 7 8 9 10+

B=BREAKFAST L=LUNCH D=DINNER S=SNACKS E=EXERCISE

HOW I FEEL

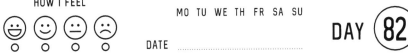

MO TU WE TH FR SA SU

DATE ....

DAY (82)

BREAKFAST

....
....
....
....
....
_____ ____

SNACKS

....
....
....

TOTAL CALORIES

_____

PROTEIN CONTENT   FIBER CONTENT

_____ _____

OTHER

....

LUNCH

....
....
....
....
....
....
....
....
....
....
....
....
_____

DINNER

....
....
....
....
....
....
....
....
....
....
....
....

WEIGHT   SLEEP   WATER   PROTEIN

_____ _____ ....

♥ EXERCISE / OTHER ACTIVITIES

	SET / REPS / DISTANCE	TIME
....	....	....
....	....	....
....	....	....
....	....	....
....	....	....

NOTES

....
....

6A 7 8 9 10 11 12P 1 2 3 4 5 6 7 8 9 10+

B=BREAKFAST   L=LUNCH   D=DINNER   S=SNACKS   E=EXERCISE

DAY (83)

MO TU WE TH FR SA SU

DATE ....

HOW I FEEL

☺ ☺ ☺ ☹
○ ○ ○ ○

BREAKFAST

....
....
....
....
....

SNACKS

....
....
....

TOTAL CALORIES

_____

PROTEIN CONTENT FIBER CONTENT

_____ _____

OTHER

....

LUNCH

....
....
....
....
....
....
....
....
....

DINNER

....
....
....
....
....
....
....
....
....

WEIGHT **SLEEP** **WATER** **PROTEIN**

....

♥ **EXERCISE / OTHER ACTIVITIES**   SET / REPS / DISTANCE   TIME

....
....
....
....
....

NOTES

....
....

🕐 6A 7 8 9 10 11 12P 1 2 3 4 5 6 7 8 9 10+

B=BREAKFAST L=LUNCH D=DINNER S=SNACKS E=EXERCISE

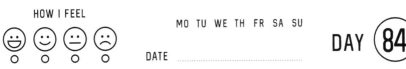

HOW I FEEL

MO TU WE TH FR SA SU

DATE ....

DAY (84)

BREAKFAST

LUNCH

DINNER

SNACKS

TOTAL CALORIES

WEIGHT

SLEEP

WATER

PROTEIN

PROTEIN CONTENT FIBER CONTENT

OTHER

♥ EXERCISE / OTHER ACTIVITIES

SET / REPS / DISTANCE

TIME

NOTES

6A 7 8 9 10 11 12P 1 2 3 4 5 6 7 8 9 10+

B=BREAKFAST L=LUNCH D=DINNER S=SNACKS E=EXERCISE

DAY (85)

MO TU WE TH FR SA SU

DATE ....

HOW I FEEL

:D :) :| :(
O   O   O   O

BREAKFAST

....
....
....
....
....
....

_____   _____

SNACKS

....
....
....
....

TOTAL CALORIES

_____

PROTEIN CONTENT FIBER CONTENT

_____   _____

OTHER

....

LUNCH

....
....
....
....
....
....
....
....
....
....

DINNER

....
....
....
....
....
....
....
....
....
....

WEIGHT   SLEEP   WATER   PROTEIN

♥ EXERCISE / OTHER ACTIVITIES

	SET / REPS / DISTANCE	TIME
....	....	....
....	....	....
....	....	....
....	....	....
....	....	....

NOTES

....
....
....

6A 7 8 9 10 11 12P 1 2 3 4 5 6 7 8 9 10+

B=BREAKFAST L=LUNCH D=DINNER S=SNACKS E=EXERCISE

HOW I FEEL

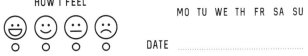

MO TU WE TH FR SA SU

DATE ....

DAY (86)

BREAKFAST
....
....
....
....
....
_____ ____

SNACKS
....
....
....
_____ ____

TOTAL CALORIES
_____

PROTEIN CONTENT FIBER CONTENT
_____ _____

OTHER
....

LUNCH
....
....
....
....
....
....
....
....
....
....

DINNER
....
....
....
....
....
....
....
....

WEIGHT   SLEEP   WATER   PROTEIN

_____ _____ ....

♥ EXERCISE / OTHER ACTIVITIES

EXERCISE / OTHER ACTIVITIES	SET / REPS / DISTANCE	TIME
....	....	....
....	....	....
....	....	....
....	....	....
....	....	....

NOTES
....
....

🕐 6A 7 8 9 10 11 12P 1 2 3 4 5 6 7 8 9 10+

B=BREAKFAST L=LUNCH D=DINNER S=SNACKS E=EXERCISE

DAY (87)

DATE ....

HOW I FEEL

😃   🙂   😐   🙁
○   ○   ○   ○

BREAKFAST

....
....
....
....
....

_____   ___

SNACKS

....
....
....

_____   ___

LUNCH

....
....
....
....
....
....
....
....
....
....

DINNER

....
....
....
....
....
....
....
....
....

TOTAL CALORIES

_____

PROTEIN CONTENT   FIBER CONTENT

_____   ___

WEIGHT   **SLEEP**   **WATER**   **PROTEIN**

OTHER ....

♥ EXERCISE / OTHER ACTIVITIES

	SET / REPS / DISTANCE	TIME
....	....	....
....	....	....
....	....	....
....	....	....
....	....	....

NOTES

....
....

🕐 6A 7 8 9 10 11 12P 1 2 3 4 5 6 7 8 9 10+

B=BREAKFAST   L=LUNCH   D=DINNER   S=SNACKS   E=EXERCISE

HOW I FEEL

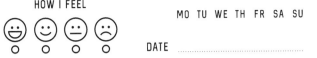

MO TU WE TH FR SA SU

DATE ....

DAY (88)

BREAKFAST
....
....
....
....
....
_____ __

SNACKS
....
....
....
_____ __

TOTAL CALORIES
_____

PROTEIN CONTENT FIBER CONTENT
_____ _____

OTHER
....

LUNCH
....
....
....
....
....
....
....
....
....
....

DINNER
....
....
....
....
....

WEIGHT   **SLEEP**   **WATER**   **PROTEIN**

....

♥ EXERCISE / OTHER ACTIVITIES   SET / REPS / DISTANCE   TIME

....
....
....
....
....

NOTES
....
....

🕐 6A 7 8 9 10 11 12P 1 2 3 4 5 6 7 8 9 10+

B=BREAKFAST L=LUNCH D=DINNER S=SNACKS E=EXERCISE

DAY (89)

MO TU WE TH FR SA SU

DATE ....

HOW I FEEL

:) :) :| :(
○ ○ ○ ○

BREAKFAST

....
....
....
....
....

SNACKS

....
....
....

TOTAL CALORIES

_____

PROTEIN CONTENT FIBER CONTENT

_____ _____

OTHER

....

LUNCH

....
....
....
....
....
....
....
....
....

DINNER

....
....
....
....
....
....
....

WEIGHT   SLEEP   WATER   PROTEIN

_____ _____ ....

♡ EXERCISE / OTHER ACTIVITIES | SET / REPS / DISTANCE | TIME

....	....	
....	....	
....	....	
....	....	
....	....	

NOTES

....
....

🕐 6A 7 8 9 10 11 12P 1 2 3 4 5 6 7 8 9 10+

B=BREAKFAST L=LUNCH D=DINNER S=SNACKS E=EXERCISE

HOW I FEEL

MO TU WE TH FR SA SU

DATE ....

DAY

BREAKFAST

....
....
....
....
....
_____ ____

SNACKS

....
....
....

TOTAL CALORIES

_____

PROTEIN CONTENT   FIBER CONTENT

_____ _____

OTHER

....

LUNCH

....
....
....
....
....
....
....
....
....
....

DINNER

....
....
....
....
....

WEIGHT   SLEEP   WATER   PROTEIN

_____ _____ ....

♥ EXERCISE / OTHER ACTIVITIES

	SET / REPS / DISTANCE	TIME
....		
....		
....		
....		
....		

NOTES

....
....

6A 7 8 9 10 11 12P 1 2 3 4 5 6 7 8 9 10+

B=BREAKFAST   L=LUNCH   D=DINNER   S=SNACKS   E=EXERCISE

DAY 90

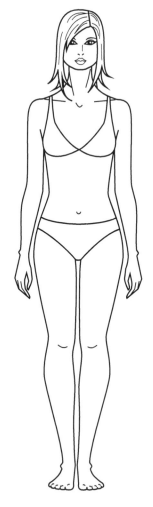

ARM ....

CHEST ....

WAIST ....

BELLY ....

HIP ....

THIGH ....

CALF ....

WEIGHT

BMI

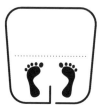

MY RESULTS

DAY 1	DAY 90		DIFFERENCE
....	....	ARM	....
....	....	CHEST	....
....	....	WAIST	....
....	....	BELLY	....
....	....	HIP	....
....	....	THIGH	....
....	....	CALF	....

WEIGHT

WEIGHT

WEIGHT

BMI

BMI

BMI

NOTES

COPYRIGHT © G.F.N. GET FIT NOTEBOOKS
PUBLISHED BY: STUDIO 5519, 1732 1ST AVE #25519 NEW YORK, NY 10128
APRIL 2017, ISSUE NO. 1 [V 1.1]: CONTACT: INFO@STUDIO5519.COM; ILLUSTRATION CREDITS: ©DEPOSITPHOTOS / @PUSHINKA11 / @GLEB_GURALNYK

41989323R00059

Printed in Poland
by Amazon Fulfillment
Poland Sp. z o.o., Wrocław